Healthy M

D0000236

Healthy Menopause

How to best manage your symptoms
and feel better than ever

LIZ EARLE

First published in Great Britain in 1995 by Boxtree Limited

This revised edition first published in 2016 by Orion Spring
An imprint of the Orion Publishing Group Ltd
Carmelite House
50 Victoria Embankment
London EC4Y 0DZ

An Hachette UK Company

1 3 5 7 9 10 8 6 4 2

Copyright © Liz Earle 1995, 2016

The moral right of Liz Earle to be identified as the author of this work has been asserted in accordance with the Copyright, Designs and Patents Act 1988.

All rights reserved. No part of this publication may be reproduced, stored in a retrieval system, or transmitted in any form or by any means, electronic, mechanical, photocopying, recording, or otherwise, without the prior permission of both the copyright owner and the above publisher of this book.

Every effort has been made to ensure that the information in this book is accurate. The information in this book will be relevant to the majority of people but may not be applicable in each individual case so it is advised that professional medical advice is obtained for specific health matters. Neither the publisher nor author accept any legal responsibility for any personal injury or other damage or loss arising from the use of the information in this book. In addition if you are concerned about your diet and exercise regime and wish to change them, you should consult a health practitioner first.

A CIP catalogue record for this book is available from the British Library.

ISBN: 978 1 4091 7566 7

Printed and bound by CPI Group (UK) Ltd, Croydon, CR0 4YY

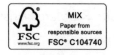

www.orionbooks.co.uk

CONTENTS

ACKNOWLEDGEMENTS

I'm grateful to Ann Bawtree and Leah Wright for helping to produce the original printed version of this book, 20 years ago, which has now been brought right up to date with the assistance of Phyllida Barnes, and Dr Louise Newson, otherwise known as the menopausedoctor.co.uk. I am also indebted to my brilliant team at Liz Earle Wellbeing for their support, as well as to my publishers at Orion and literary agent, Rosemary Sandberg. Many thanks for everyone's unfailing enthusiasm and support for such an important subject.

www.lizearlewellbeing.com

Introduction

The menopause, also known as 'the Change' and in some medical circles as the 'Climacteric', affects almost all women at some point during our lifetime. It's a natural stage in our lives but still something that is not often talked about in much detail, or openly, and lots of women know very little about it until they experience it themselves.

Many women don't realise just how the menopause may adversely affect their lives, both at home and at work. The symptoms can start suddenly – and come as a bit of a shock. And often, because sometimes symptoms are not openly discussed, we may not even be aware that it might be the menopause causing them and that, in the great majority of cases, they can be treated easily, effectively and safely.

All menopause symptoms are caused by fluctuating, low or no levels of hormones and the hormone treatments (HRT) that are available to women now are very much safer than many may think, and much more naturally derived and 'body identical' than preparations used in the past. HRT can both improve our menopausal symptoms and help reduce our increased risk of heart disease and osteoporosis. So it's a subject that's well worth exploring.

There are also a few non-hormone and complementary treatments and therapies available which can sometimes ease some of the symptoms. A combination of these treatments, plus greater nutritional knowledge and our awareness of both the power of exercise, good nutrition and open, frank discussion, can enable the menopause to be an event in our lives that can be embraced and fully prepared for. This quick guide sets out practical, impartial and well-rounded advice and information to help all of us either approaching or in the midst of their menopause – and I really hope it will enable you to better cope with and enjoy this phase of your life.

A few simple shifts in the way we think about our health, our attitude, much more openness about the subject, and simple changes to diet and lifestyle will help all of us going through the menopause to better equip ourselves to enjoy life to the full during this time of natural – and eventually rewarding – change. The best personal advice I can give is, 'Keep talking – to your friends and also your GP if necessary' (see MANAGING YOUR MENOPAUSE AND THE IMPORTANCE OF FRIENDSHIP, pages 54–7). A problem confronted and shared is very often a problem halved or solved and it's always reassuring to know that you're not the only woman suffering with a symptom – especially one that you'll find is very common in your age group – and for which there will almost certainly be a solution or a treatment. Wishing you a happy, healthy and stress-free menopause!

Liz Earle MBE

– 1 –

The Menopause

There are so many major changes that occur during our lives; from teenage years, leaving home, careers, relationships and sometimes marriage and motherhood. The menopause – also known as the Change or the Climacteric – is another of life's milestones and with knowledge, care and (if you need it) professional help, it really needn't be feared or dreaded. It fact, in some ways it can even be embraced as the beginning of a new and exciting phase of life.

So why the dread? In days gone by the onset of menstruation was something to be feared. There were many scare stories of what a girl could expect and how restricted her life would become during 'those days' each month. Now, monthly sanitary protection is advertised all around us in the Western world – often very bluntly, pulling no punches with vocabulary, sometimes even using images that portray blood and showing menstruating women as strong, determined and beautiful. We know full well that a woman's life does not come to a full stop one week in every four, and we take steps to ensure that this is the case, too.

So why is it that menopausal women often do not share this same positive image or attitude? Possibly because the menopause is not often openly discussed and its symptoms are frequently secret, ignored, not dealt with properly or maybe not even recognised as being menopause related. A very common attitude is: 'This is a natural process therefore I will put up with it and wait till it's over.' But these symptoms of a natural process could take 10 years or longer to be over and may interfere negatively with your life, so it's well worth dealing with them sooner rather than later and giving yourself the chance to have a happy, healthy and productive 'change of life'.

There's still a fear coupled with acceptance that the menopause is a time when women have to suffer hot flushes, cold sweats, headaches, indecisiveness, depression, vaginal dryness and mood swings for over a decade until they finally fall into a grey-haired, incontinent heap of disintegrating bones. However, we only have to look around us to see that this is just not true. Many menopausal women are confident, happy, fulfilled and absolutely delighted to 'be themselves' – often living a bit more for themselves, possibly after decades of concentrated caring for children or parents or doing a demanding job. Or they might be at the pinnacle of their career and/or lives as mothers, taking great pleasure in whatever they are doing. They are likely to be either the one in five women who suffer no negative menopausal symptoms or the ones who have sought and found workable solutions to make life easier.

And of course there are millions of post-menopausal women living happy, fulfilled and healthy lives with the added advantage of not having to worry about unintended pregnancy; they are often very comfortable with their own sexuality and what it takes for them to have a fulfilling sex life.

In the twenty-first century, the message of some in the Western world is that in order to be beautiful it is necessary to be young. Isn't it therefore only logical to believe that to be old is to be unattractive? Are signs of ageing any cause for dismay? No, it's obviously possible to be post-menopausal and beautiful, even into advanced old age, especially if we exercise regularly, eat well and keep challenging ourselves to learn more, see more and continue taking an interest and engaging in the wider world. One of the joys of middle age is the ability and freedom to really 'be oneself', coupled with the growing certainty that life is finite and therefore really to be enjoyed, a day at a time, with few regrets, living in the moment. An older woman with wisdom and confidence who has survived the challenges of a career, possibly marriage and possibly motherhood, is almost always an attractive and interesting person to spend time with. She usually has a confidence grown from experiences enjoyed or survived and a wry take on the world that is compelling and reassuring for younger people. No, youth does not equal beauty any more than fertility is the same as femininity, and this time of life is a good moment to take stock and begin to appreciate who you have become and what you may still achieve and do – or even change.

It's well worth remembering at this point that at the beginning of the twentieth century – in 1916 – life expectancy for women was 56.5 years, meaning that many women then either didn't reach the menopause or had a very short menopause. The huge majority of us now will reach our menopause and some of us will live with and then after it for often 30–40 years. So it is well worth being aware of the symptoms and how they may affect you, and of course knowing how to deal with them in as quick and as efficient a way as possible. We have busy lives that require energy and creativity so why would we want to do otherwise?

WHAT IS THE MENOPAUSE?

The word menopause actually means your last menstrual period (*Meno-* means menstrual and *-pause* refers to stop). The menopause occurs when your ovaries stop producing eggs and as a result of this the levels of your hormones – mainly oestrogen and progesterone – fall.

The changes that accompany the menopause do not usually occur suddenly, but develop over a number of years. We all change throughout our lives and many of these changes are brought about by our hormones. These are natural chemicals made by various glands in the body which are released into our bloodstream. Each month, hormones are made by the pituitary gland in your brain and are released into your bloodstream to prompt your ovaries to produce oestrogen and progesterone. Oestrogen and progesterone are responsible for puberty, but these two hormones also have the important job of preparing the lining of the womb to receive a fertilised egg, so that it can grow into a baby. If no egg arrives, this lining is shed and is then lost in the flow of menstrual blood. After a few days the monthly process restarts. At the menopause this regular monthly cycle stops.

Oestrogen also protects a number of different systems in your body; for example, your brain, bones, heart, skin, hair and vagina, so low levels can affect many different areas of your body.

You also have testosterone in your body, which is an important hormone. Many may think of testosterone as the 'male' hormone, which is correct, but we need to have testosterone too. In fact, surprisingly, women produce three times as much testosterone as oestrogen before their menopause. Testosterone is made in our ovaries and also in our adrenal glands, which are small glands near the kidneys. Testosterone helps maintain muscle and bone mass in women and contributes to sex drive. It also helps with mood, energy and concentration. Levels of testosterone in our body gradually reduce as we become older or when our ovaries stop working.

A woman is referred to as being menopausal when her last menstrual period was one year ago. Many women have very irregular and often scanty periods before they finally stop their periods, so in practice the term perimenopause is more often used. This is the time in which you experience menopausal symptoms but are still having periods. The hormones oestrogen and progesterone work together to regulate your menstrual cycle and also the production of eggs. During your perimenopause the levels of these hormones fluctuate and it is often the imbalance of these hormones which leads to symptoms of the menopause occurring.

The perimenopause (the transition to menopause) usually starts in a woman's forties and lasts until her menopause. The term pre-menopause is usually used to describe the time in your life before any symptoms of the menopause occur and the term post-menopause is used to describe the time in your life after your menopause.

The average age at which women experience their menopause in the UK is 51 years, however, this can be earlier for some women. Symptoms of the perimenopause often start at around 45 years of age. If the menopause occurs before the age of 40 it is classed as Premature Ovarian Insufficiency (POI). If the menopause occurs when a woman is under 45 years of age then it is classed as an early menopause.

Although the menopause is a normal event in a woman's lifetime, certain conditions and medical procedures can bring about an early menopause. These include having your ovaries removed during an operation, having radiotherapy to your pelvic area as a treatment for cancer or receiving certain types of chemotherapy drugs that treat cancer. All these can cause an early menopause.

If you have had your womb (uterus) removed (an operation called a hysterectomy) before your menopause, you may experience an early menopause, even if your ovaries are not removed. Although your ovaries will still make some oestrogen after your hysterectomy, it is common that your level of oestrogen will fall at an earlier age than average. As you don't have periods after a hysterectomy, it may not be clear when you are in the menopause. However, you may develop some typical symptoms (see SYMPTOMS OF THE MENOPAUSE AND HOW TO DEAL WITH THEM, pages 22–47) when your oestrogen level falls.

An early menopause runs in some families, so it's worth discussing this with your parents and other relations in case this is relevant to you, so that you are aware of this possibility and can get medical help if and when you need it. (See EARLY MENOPAUSE AND PREMATURE OVARIAN INSUFFICIENCY, pages 13–14.)

The length of time that menopausal symptoms lasts for varies tremendously between women. Encouragingly, around one in five women do not have any symptoms at all.

However, the vast majority of women do have symptoms, with around one in four having severe symptoms that really affect the quality of their lives. Some women only have symptoms for a few years (two to five years) but around 10–20 per cent of women experience them for longer than 10 years. Some women even have hot flushes in their eighties!

After the menopause you are no longer fertile. The current recommendations are that if you are under 50 years of age when your periods stop you should continue with contraception for two years, whereas if you are 50 years or over you only need to continue with contraception for another year after your last period.

Taking the combined contraceptive pill may mask the menopause by controlling menopausal symptoms such as hot flushes and night sweats. It may therefore be difficult to tell when you are no longer fertile. So you must continue with contraception if you are not keen on a late, unplanned pregnancy; there are many stories of women believing they are entering the menopause (and they may well be) only to find that they are pregnant – myself included at the age of 47!

– 2 –

How the Menopause
is Diagnosed

If you are over 45 years old and have irregular periods with symptoms of the menopause, then you don't need to have any tests to diagnose the menopause. If you are taking contraception or have a Mirena coil, it may be difficult to know what your periods are like. However, if you are having symptoms of the menopause and are over 45 years of age you do not need blood tests either. The diagnosis is made purely on your symptoms and your age.

If you're under 45 and are experiencing symptoms, it might be worth asking your GP for a blood test. The most common one is a blood test measuring the level of a hormone called follicle-stimulating hormone (FSH). This is the hormone that regulates the amount of oestrogen in your body. If you have low levels of oestrogen in your body your FSH level is usually raised. If this is raised, then it is very likely that you are menopausal or perimenopausal. This blood test is often repeated four to six weeks later. However, as your hormone levels fluctuate some women have a normal FSH level and are still menopausal or perimenopausal. You should certainly not be told you are or are not menopausal or perimenopausal by just one blood test if you are under 45 years old.

If you are under 40 years of age you may be advised to have other blood tests in addition to FSH levels, for example some types of genetic tests. Some women may also be recommended to have a bone density test (DEXA scan) to determine the strength of their bones.

– 3 –

Early Menopause and Premature Ovarian Insufficiency (POI)

Premature Ovarian Insufficiency (POI) is when your ovaries stop working properly before the age of 40. Here, your ovaries often do not necessarily completely fail, which is different to the menopause. This means that the function of your ovaries can fluctuate over time, occasionally resulting in a period, ovulation or even pregnancy, sometimes several years after diagnosis. This temporary working of the ovaries means that around 5–10 per cent of women with POI are able to conceive.

Although most women with POI have symptoms of the menopause, around one in four don't experience any symptoms of the menopause at all other than having irregular or no periods. The most common way of diagnosing POI is by having a blood test. So do talk to your GP if this is a concern.

This is a very important condition to diagnose promptly as without treatment, in the form of hormones, there is a greater risk of developing conditions such as osteoporosis and heart attacks. According to menopause expert Dr Louise Newson, it's very important if you're diagnosed with POI that you receive hormones (HRT or the contraceptive pill) up to the natural age of menopause (51 years) to replace the hormones that your body would otherwise be producing. There are **no risks** attached to taking HRT when you are young and Dr Newson maintains that it is completely safe to take. This is because you are replacing the hormones that your body should otherwise be producing.

– 4 –

Contraception
for the Over-40s

Thanks to organisations such as Women's Health Concern (WHC), which is part of the British Menopause Society, we all have access to good, unbiased advice on many of the specific sexual health issues we might be bothered by during the menopause, one of which is contraception. WHC has many useful factsheets on their website (womens-health-concern. org) including advice on contraception for older women. As does the Faculty of Sexual & Reproductive Healthcare of the Royal College of Obstetricians & Gynaecologists. (See USEFUL CONTACTS, page 101, for more information.)

It's worth repeating that current recommendations are that if you're under 50 years of age when your periods stop, then you should continue with contraception for two years, whereas if you are 50 years or over you only need to continue with contraception for another year after your last period.

Because some hormonal methods of contraception can

also be helpful in reducing symptoms of the menopause, I've also included some information on this here.

HORMONAL METHODS

The combined pill

Studies show that the combined pill can safely be used until the age of 50, as long as there are no health risks, such as smoking, obesity, high blood pressure, etc., that could lead to stroke or heart or blood-clotting problems. Your local doctor or nurse will be able to advise on this.

The pill has several advantages for women in this age group as it also regulates periods, may help to maintain bone mineral density (which is reduced after the menopause), may reduce blood loss and period pains and may also relieve some of the more troublesome menopausal symptoms, such as hot flushes and night sweats.

The contraceptive patch and vaginal ring

The efficacy, benefits, risks and side-effects of these methods are similar to the combined pill and again it can be safely prescribed until 50 years old to those with no health risks.

PROGESTOGEN-ONLY METHODS

All progestogen-only methods may cause irregular bleeding or even no bleeding at all. The absence of bleeding doesn't necessarily mean that the menopause has been reached, it is just a side-effect of the method of contraception. Do check back with your GP if bleeding occurs after a long time with no periods.

The progestogen-only pill (POP or mini-pill)

The progestogen-only pill is suitable for older women and can safely be used up until the age of 55.

The contraceptive injection

It's recommended that use of this method can continue until the age of 50. There has been some concern that the injection may reduce bone mineral density and increase the risk of osteoporosis. So those with a lifestyle or risk factors for osteoporosis (smokers, previous fractures, steroid use, family history, etc.) may wish to think about another method of contraception.

Contraceptive implants

The implant is suitable until the age of 50 and there are no anxieties about loss of bone mineral density with this method.

Intrauterine system (IUS)

The hormone-releasing IUS (usually a Mirena coil) is not only a highly effective method of contraception but it also significantly reduces the amount of bleeding and period pain. This is particularly important as a considerable number of women complain of heavy periods and 'flooding' in their forties. Also, if a woman decides to start HRT during the perimenopause, then the IUS can be used as the progestogen element of HRT, which can be handy as you then don't have to worry about taking daily progesterone.

The IUS is licensed for contraception for five years. It can be used as the progesterone part of HRT also for five years.

The Faculty of Sexual and Reproductive Healthcare of the Royal College of Obstetricians and Gynaecologists has a website with links to current clinical guidance regarding contraception in women over 40 years and, of course, you should discuss options with your GP. Do check it out for the latest recommendations and updates in this important area.

– 5 –

Why is it so Important to Deal with the Symptoms of the Menopause?

The average age of the menopause is now 51 years; advances in our hygiene, medicine and, for many, improved nutrition and lifestyle means that our life expectancy is around 82 years in the UK. That's a big jump (hoorah!) and also means that we are likely to spend around a third of our lives being post-menopausal. We women obviously want to enjoy our lives as we become older and to try to ensure our future health and wellbeing is as good as possible. Ensuring that your menopause does not interfere with your quality of life is really important; your life could be long and many of us who are approaching or experiencing our menopause now could still be working and caring for others well past what has until recently been considered retirement age! We need to be confident that our fluctuating hormone levels aren't adversely affecting either us or the people around us.

The menopause often occurs at a difficult time in life. You may feel age-related pressures at work or within your relationship. If you have them, your children may be leaving home or your relatives may be older and losing some of their independence and relying on you for help more and more. Financial pressures may also be great, with children now needing financial support often until their mid-twenties and beyond. Whether you are single, married, divorced or have a partner, these pressures can obviously lead to many emotional changes and you might not recognise that some of these are actually related to your menopause and can be medically helped. As Dr Louann Brizendine, the author of *The Female Brain* says,

> The mummy brain unplugs. Menopause means a lowering of the hormones that have boosted communication circuits, emotion circuits, the drive to tend and care, and the urge to avoid conflict at all costs.

It is helpful to know that sometimes our bodies may be driving us to make decisions that, were our hormones in better balance, we might consider to be unhelpful in the long term. We may become short-tempered or feel less caring towards those in our family. And it's another reason to nurture your friendships so that the people who know you best can help you through the tricky patches that are inevitable in most of our lives. Take time to keep long-standing relationships and friendships alive.

The other, relatively recent, change is that because many women now give birth on average later than in previous generations, they may experience their menopause at the time when their own children are either very young or adolescent; the consequent heady mix of fluctuating hormones and conflicting needs in a household is a very common conversation topic nowadays – especially among those around me!

Women feel very differently regarding their own menopause. The menopause is a personal experience and women deal with the psychological aspects of it in very different ways. You may very much enjoy not having periods any more but the menopause clearly affects your fertility. For women who've completed their family, or who don't want children, this can be a relief. But for younger women, especially those with Premature Ovarian Insufficiency (POI), an early menopause can be associated with reduced fertility which often leads to many psychological problems, such as stress, anxiety and lack of confidence.

− 6 −

Symptoms of the Menopause and How to Deal with Them

The menopause is a natural event for all women. You may have no problems at all and simply notice that your periods have stopped. However, if you are reading this book that is perhaps less likely. Menopausal symptoms vary tremendously between us; some will only experience them for a few months while others can continue to suffer with symptoms for many years, even after their last period.

Some of these symptoms may have a negative effect on your other half, your family, your work colleagues and your life in general. It's common for symptoms to come and go, so you may have some months where you feel completely fine and then other times when you experience unpleasant symptoms which adversely affect the quality of your life and are emotionally very lowering.

Around half of women going through the Change say their symptoms are worse than they had anticipated. Hormones rule so much of our lives at this time. Oestrogen is actually mainly three different hormones: oestradiol, oestrone and oestriol. Oestrogen itself has over 300 functions in maintaining the health of our skin, muscles, hair, digestion, brain and more, so it is not surprising that when they are unbalanced, our body is also in a highly sensitive, delicate and reactive state.

CHANGE IN YOUR MENSTRUAL CYCLE

The first sign of the menopause is usually a change in your menstrual cycle. This may be irregular periods – happening more or less often – or your periods being lighter or even much heavier. All women will experience a change to their menstrual cycle when they are perimenopausal or menopausal.

HOT FLUSHES

The most common symptoms of the menopause are hot flushes and night sweats. Hot flushes occur in around three out of four women. They usually come on very suddenly and often spread throughout your body, chest, neck and face. They vary in length from a few minutes to much longer. Women who have hot flushes report everything from a sudden warm feeling to a sensation of tremendous heat and being bathed in perspiration. They often happen at night and can wake you up, causing sleep disturbance, which is a problem in itself.

Hot flushes can be associated with symptoms such as sweating, dizziness, light-headedness and even heart palpitations. They may happen many times throughout the day and can go on for many years. They can vary from occurring very occasionally to once or twice a day or one every hour. They usually occur spontaneously and are very unpredictable. However, they can also happen after eating certain types of food, such as hot, spicy food, or drinking alcohol, especially wine. Women who smoke are more likely to have more severe and more frequent hot flushes.

Hot flushes are thought to be due to the low levels of oestrogen in your body affecting a part of our brain called the hypothalamus. The hypothalamus regulates body temperature; the decrease in oestrogen in our body affects how our hypothalamus works and it inaccurately senses that your body is overheating. This leads to blood vessels dilating (becoming larger), allowing more blood to flow to the skin, causing it to redden and heat up. Often our brain then registers that it has overdone it and so switches on perspiration to cool down the overheated areas. This gives rise to anything from a slight clamminess to rivers of sweat; this is obviously sometimes extremely socially awkward.

Stopping smoking and cutting down your alcohol intake – or even stopping drinking alcohol or switching from wine to an occasional vodka (considered the purest form of spirits) – can often help to reduce the number and severity of hot flushes. Some women experience heart palpitations with their hot flushes. These can be both caused and exacerbated by alcohol so if you are affected, it's sensible to avoid alcohol as much as possible. You might sleep much better, too! The same pulse-raising effects apply to caffeine; coffee, tea, dark chocolate, some fizzy drinks and even certain painkillers (check ingredients on common painkillers and fizzy drinks if you are sensitive to caffeine) contain caffeine. Cutting out caffeine in the afternoon is also often beneficial. It's important to drink plenty of water as this both helps your body stay cool and also replaces water you may have lost when having a hot flush.

Interestingly, hot flushes do not occur in every society and are generally more common in the developed West than in the East and some developing countries. In some of these countries women are not bothered by these symptoms, and in Japan there is not even a word for hot flushes. Some research suggests that soy, a significant element of the Japanese diet, may be useful in preventing hot flushes in women. Edible beans, especially soya beans, contain the compounds genistein and daidzein, which are oestrogenic and can help to control hot flushes. Cooking soy-rich foods, such as replacing conventional flour with soya flour in recipes, may be helpful and I talk more about this towards the end of the book (see page 85).

NIGHT SWEATS

Night sweats are also very common and very troublesome. They're thought to be caused by the same mechanism that causes hot flushes. Many women find they wake up several times each night and are 'drenched' with sweat, so much so that they need to change their bed clothes and bed linen. This is obviously very disruptive for anyone else in the bedroom, too.

Wearing cotton or bamboo-fibre clothing rather than man-made, synthetic fibres can be helpful as natural materials allow our skin to 'breathe' more and are cooler than synthetic fibres. In cool weather, several layers of easily removable lightweight clothing are better than woollens, as it's easier to adjust them if you feel a hot flush coming on . . . Having a constant supply of water with you and also having a small fan can be very useful.

Cotton or linen sheets and duvet covers are better than a cotton/polyester mix in dealing with sweating at night. The tight weave on a thread count of more than 120 traps heat, causing the 'covers-on covers-off' game that is characteristic of menopausal nights. Opt for low thread-count cotton, or better still, long-lasting linen – which has a thread count of 80–150 and better wicking properties, meaning less fluctuation in temperature and a less interrupted night's sleep. If you sleep with a partner, it might be a good time to invest in separate duvets, taking into account your individual heating/cooling needs. Common in European countries, this is actually a very handy tip.

Never leave the heating on all night and, if you can, introduce a movement of air in the bedroom – perhaps by opening a window or a door. Water and facial tonic spritzers can also be helpful; let the mist evaporate on your skin for maximum coolness. Keep a spritz beside the bed.

MOOD SWINGS, DEPRESSION AND PSYCHOLOGICAL PROBLEMS

Unfortunately, mood swings are common, too, and you may find that your mood is more unpredictable than it used to be. Your low oestrogen levels influence the production of serotonin in your body, a chemical that helps to regulate our mood. You may find that your mood fluctuates considerably without any triggers or any obvious reason and sometimes find yourself weeping at times and in situations that really surprise you. We may also find ourselves short-tempered or less tolerant of those around us. This is natural – if unhelpful!

Mood swings are more likely if you have had premenstrual syndrome (PMS) in the past. Some of us find that our PMS symptoms, such as bloating, irritability, food cravings, mood swings and lethargy, worsen. These symptoms are usually due to the fluctuating levels of progesterone in the body.

Emotional symptoms during the perimenopause and menopause vary greatly between women. Some women find that symptoms of depression, anxiety, panic attacks, anger and irritation worsen so much that they really interfere with the quality of their life. These symptoms can affect your emotional wellbeing and significantly increase the stress of life in general.

Eating well and regularly, cutting down on alcohol and caffeine, exercising regularly doing activities or sports that you enjoy, making time for your friends and taking time out – maybe by walking and talking, treating yourself to a massage possibly with aromatherapy, investing in some acupuncture or going to a yoga or exercise class – are all things you can do yourself to minimise mood swings and emotional symptoms and help put things into perspective. It's important to make time for these non-work, me-time things. Often our responsibilities are huge at this time of life and coping with them constructively means valuing and looking after yourself – sometimes the person who is managing many aspects of your own and your family's or colleagues' lives all at once – properly.

TIREDNESS AND POOR SLEEP

Tiredness can easily be a consequence of disrupted sleep from night sweats and possibly palpitations. However, even without these symptoms, many women find that they have a more unsettled and less fulfilling night's sleep when they are perimenopausal. Even if your sleep is not affected, you may find that you are more tired than normal during the day. This tiredness can be overwhelming and can really affect your ability to function properly in the daytime. Sometimes this is due to low levels of testosterone.

Going to bed at roughly the same time of night every night and switching off all screens a good hour before you need to sleep is a good practical way of minimising sleep disruption. This is because the light rays emitted from screens has been shown to disrupt the pituitary gland that controls sleep. Buying a blue filter cover to fit over your smartphone or tablet screen can be helpful if you can't put your gadget down, as this reduces the gland-disrupting glare. It can also be helpful to drink less or no alcohol and no caffeinated drinks in the afternoon. A cup of chamomile or valerian tea last thing at night might also encourage a better night's sleep. A cup of coffee almost definitely won't!

If you can't live without hot drinks, there are so many fantastic herbal and fruit teas available, or you can make your own from fresh herbs, such as mint leaves and/or fennel fronds. Or, if you really want to drink tea or coffee in the late afternoon or evening, choose decaffeinated versions.

LACK OF LIBIDO

Reduced or absent libido (sex drive) can occur when your hormone levels fall. We still don't know exactly which combination and levels of hormones will maintain a woman's libido, but it's fair to say that many women find that they desire sex less as they age and that sex can be less pleasurable than it used to be.

Lack of libido also happens when life is incredibly busy and demanding; maybe you and your partner aren't making time for each other or yourselves and all you need to do is plan a special night away or evening out, where you aren't at home or work and faced with all your responsibilities. It's really important to do this because, as I've said before, the menopause often occurs at a time when you have lots of responsibilities and it's easy to ignore relationships. I can't exaggerate the importance of maintaining both your friendships and family relationships; they are like most plants and need nurturing.

Sometimes a lack of libido will be due to another very common menopausal symptom; dryness of the vagina, which can be due to a lack of oestrogen. A dry vagina can also be caused by medications such as anti-depressants and some cold and allergy medicines. This can cause discomfort during sex, which will probably put you off the whole idea, and your libido will be lowered. It's a vicious cycle. This dryness is usually dealt with easily and – of course – breaking the cycle can lead to a return of libido. This is an important topic for many women and an important factor in many relationships, so I've devoted a whole section to it (see SOLUTIONS AND TREATMENTS FOR VAGINAL DRYNESS, pages 77–80).

If both investing time in your sexual relationship and dealing with vaginal dryness doesn't increase your libido, it may be helpful to discuss your potential need for testosterone with your GP.

URINARY INCONTINENCE

Few things are as disheartening as finding your bladder is no longer completely in your control. Not being able to bounce on a trampoline with your children or play your sport of choice, having to consider carefully what you wear and finding yourself with a couple of packs of sanitary pads in your shopping trolley on a regular basis are all things guaranteed to lower your spirit. Incontinence can range from a slight spurt when you sneeze to truly wetting yourself if you are unable to get to a loo immediately when you first feel the need. These typify two different types of incontinence: stress incontinence and urge incontinence. Although urinary incontinence is hardly ever spoken about, both types are in fact very, very common and, fortunately, very treatable. It's a condition that is more common during and after the menopause.

In addition to these symptoms, some women notice that their pelvic floor muscles weaken when they go through the menopause. This can result in feeling you need to pass urine more frequently and finding it more difficult to 'hold onto' your bowel or bladder.

Your kidneys make urine continuously. A trickle of urine is constantly passing to your bladder down your ureters (the tubes from your kidneys to your bladder). We make different amounts of urine depending on how much we drink, eat and perspire.

Our bladder is made of muscle and stores urine, expanding like a balloon as it fills. The outlet for urine (the urethra) is normally kept closed by pelvic floor muscles. The pelvic floor muscles are in a sling shape from the back of the pubic bone at the front, to the front of the base of the spine at the back. These muscles usually work without us even thinking about them, supporting our pelvic organs, bladder and womb, and controlling the passage of urine.

When a certain volume of urine is in our bladders, we become aware that the bladder is getting full. Then when we go to the loo, our bladder muscle squeezes (contracts) and our urethra and pelvic floor muscles relax to allow the urine to flow out. There are complex nerve messages between our brain, bladder and pelvic floor muscles which work to tell us how full the bladder is and also to tell the correct muscles to contract or relax at the right time.

Stress incontinence
The muscles and tissues which support our bladder can become weaker with the passage of time. Many factors contribute to this and they include childbearing, constipation, being overweight or obese and the general lessening of muscle tone that is caused by lack of oestrogen.

Pelvic floor muscles can become weak or damaged, particularly during childbirth, so that they are then less effective at supporting the pelvic organs or controlling the passage of urine. Stress incontinence means that we leak urine at times when there is an increase of pressure on our bladder – for example when we sneeze, cough or jump. Stress incontinence is the most common type of urinary incontinence and occurs in at least one in five women over the age of 40.

There are different treatments available for stress incontinence and for most women these lead to a cure or a marked improvement in their symptoms. To prevent stress incontinence, we need to strengthen our pelvic muscles by very regular pelvic floor exercises – particularly Kegel exercises – which can improve the support of your pelvic organs and the control of urine. These exercises should become part of your daily routine – for life. Ideally they should be started in our twenties and always after giving birth. If you have daughters, nieces or goddaughters then you should tell them about these exercises, too, so that they can get started on them early! (See BLADDER MATTERS in USEFUL CONTACTS, page 101, for detailed advice on pelvic floor exercises.)

You do need to be very motivated and disciplined to do these exercises. It can take a few months before you notice any benefit from them but you will be forever grateful if you do invest enough time and effort in them. Being completely continent is also a great plus in the sex department, as worrying about one's personal hygiene can, of course, also lower your libido. Get going on the exercises as soon and as often as you possibly can – there's even a helpful NHS app called Squeezy which will discretely remind you to 'squeeze' in the right way throughout the day!

Your doctor may refer you to a specialist physiotherapist or a continence advisor who may suggest other treatments in addition to the pelvic floor exercises. These may include using vaginal cones, which are small plastic cones that you insert into your vagina and which help you to exercise your pelvic floor muscles in a very targeted way. These come in different weights and you will progress to using heavier weights as your pelvic floor muscles strengthen. There are other devices that can really help which may also be offered to you. A trip to a women's physio is likely to reap valuable rewards.

If these treatments don't work or don't help enough, you may be offered an operation. There are many different operations available and your doctor will be able to discuss the most appropriate one for you in detail. If surgery is not an option for you, medication can sometimes be given, which can work well. Vaginal ring pessaries are also available, which support your internal organs. These are often used for women who cannot have or don't want an operation. They can be very effective and are left in usually for a year before they are replaced by your doctor. You can still have sexual intercourse with them in place. HRT can also help this kind of incontinence in the way that it helps all other kinds of muscles, as the oestrogen can help to improve your pelvic floor muscle tone, too.

Urge incontinence

Urge incontinence occurs when you cannot reach the loo quickly enough because you don't have enough warning before needing to empty your bladder. You may find that you need to pass urine more frequently and even need to get up more often in the night to do so. Urge incontinence can be caused by infection, destruction of the nerves controlling your bladder, or thinning of the tissues of the tubing along which your urine flows. Some women have a combination of stress and urge incontinence.

Urge incontinence is usually due to an overactive bladder. This means that your bladder does not fill up properly and tells your brain that you need to empty your bladder even when it is not full. You may find that you need to pass urine more frequently when you are stressed.

Drinks containing caffeine (such as tea, coffee and cola) can irritate the lining of your bladder and make urge incontinence worse. Other drinks, such as fruit juices, can also irritate your bladder, especially first thing in the morning when hitting an empty system. It's worth making your first drink of the day a glass of water (hot or cold), to rehydrate the body and settle the bladder in gently, before hitting it with a cup of tea, coffee or orange juice. A simple switch – but it works.

Having low levels of oestrogen can also affect the lining of your bladder and your urethra, which will often contribute to and worsen these symptoms. Other conditions can cause urge incontinence, too. For example, having a urinary tract infection, or a condition that affects nerves, such as multiple sclerosis or Parkinson's disease.

There are different treatments for urge incontinence and sometimes you may be advised to follow a combination of these. Reducing or even stopping caffeine intake is very important. Reducing your alcohol intake can also be beneficial. It's important to drink plenty of fluids; if you don't, this can lead to concentrated urine being produced which will irritate the lining of your bladder and make your symptoms worse.

Trying to go to the loo less frequently can work to 'retrain' your bladder and is effective for some women. Your physiotherapy or continence advisor will be able to make a personal action plan for you.

If these simple measures don't help, there are different types of medication that can work really well. If the one you are prescribed doesn't work, you may be offered another which may be more effective. If medication doesn't help, there are different operations which may be offered to you, depending on the cause and severity of your symptoms.

INCREASED STOMACH GAS

Another symptom of the menopause that causes distress and surprise is passing wind more, which occurs as a result of having increased stomach gas while perimenopausal. It may be just about tolerable if you are settled into a long and comfortable marriage or partnership, but it is very unwelcome if you are newly dating, thinking about dating or otherwise exposed to situations (such as at work), when this symptom might be really tricky. Two-thirds of women report that they experience increased stomach gas during menopause, according to a survey conducted by the Market Research Institute – so you're not alone!

Strictly speaking, the increase in stomach gas occurs during perimenopause because the balance of the bacteria involved in the digestive process is disturbed by the fluctuating and changing levels of oestrogen and progesterone.

Your intestines contain 'good bacteria' and 'bad bacteria'. Both are necessary for optimal digestion. When the good and bad bacteria are in balance, healthy digestion occurs. When the balance between good and bad bacteria is upset (an increase in bad bacteria), the digestive patterns of the body are altered, resulting in an increase in the production of gas during menopause. The most effective way to relieve excess stomach gas caused by changing levels of oestrogen and progesterone is to balance the levels of both these hormones. However, doing the following may also help reduce your stomach gas:

- Eating smaller portions of food more frequently (eating large portions less often can lower digestive function).

- Chewing your food more slowly. This will break the food into smaller chunks and allow the digestive enzymes in your saliva to do their work efficiently. Chew each mouthful 20–30 times before swallowing.

- Many of the foods (beans, lentils, wholewheat flour, etc.) that may help reduce your other symptoms of the menopause are great gas-encouragers! So if you are really struggling with excess gas, it might be a good idea to cut down a bit on these well-known culprits.

- Eat more gut-friendly foods, including plain live yoghurt (homemade is inexpensive and very easy) and kefir (a super-yoghurt drink brimming with beneficial bacteria). Read more on this in my bestseller *The Good Gut Guide* (Orion Spring).

- Take a probiotic supplement to boost the levels of beneficial gut bacteria – which is helpful for all-round good health in any case. Choose a capsule or powder that contains several different strains of beneficial micro-flora, look online for those with at least 6–10 varieties.

- Exercise regularly. Exercise increases the flow of blood through your body. This stimulates your digestive system and helps it to work more efficiently. Increased gas during menopause is much more prevalent in sedentary women and being active improves this symptom as well as just about every other.

POOR CONCENTRATION AND MEMORY

Short-term memory loss has become a bit of a running joke when it comes to menopausal women and it's common to find that you don't concentrate as well as you used to. Many of us find it harder to multitask (the thing we are traditionally so good at!) which can be so very frustrating. Many women describe having a 'brain fog', where they find it really hard to think clearly and sensibly. This can be very worrying if you're not aware that this can be connected to the menopause – and it is a very common symptom.

Many women find they forget words, names, birthdays and even do annoyingly silly things (forgetting where you parked the car 20 minutes before, putting your purse in the freezer or forgetting appointments are common examples of this!). Many women find that their brain doesn't feel as engaged as it used to and this can really affect your ability to work and function. It also causes worry; 'Why can I not think straight or remember everything I have to do? What is wrong with me?'

While we know that drops in hormone levels may contribute to this perceived lack of concentration and memory, it is good and reassuring to remember, again, that this often coincides with an incredibly busy time of life for many of us: having a responsible job, caring and/or parenting commitments and possibly volunteering and community projects. Don't be too hard on yourself and do keep talking to your friends. If nothing else, you will share some pretty funny stories . . .

JOINT PAINS AND STIFFNESS

Oestrogen is very important in providing lubrication and reducing inflammation in your joints. Low levels of oestrogen can lead to many of our joints feeling stiff and aching, particularly first thing in the morning. This may affect the way that you exercise, which can be frustrating. It can also make you feel as though you are 'very old' or as if you have arthritis or another illness that is not 'just the menopause', and again, this can be worrying. Also, on some days you may feel 25 and on others 75; this is normal for some menopausal women, but of course frustrating. Talk to your GP if you are worried. Do keep moving and exercising. Running, walking, yoga, Pilates, Zumba, tennis, golf and swimming as well as any sport that you enjoy are all fantastically good ways to keep you healthy and positive, as long as you still get pleasure from them. They also help keep your bones strong (see OSTEOPOROSIS, pages 48–51).

SKIN CHANGES

Although our skin changes as we get older, often because of exposure to the sun and wind and pollutants, as well as genetics, the changes in our hormone levels can also contribute to this. Oestrogen is important for building collagen, the protein that supports the structure of our skin. Lower levels of oestrogen can lead to reduced elasticity of our skin, dry skin, fine lines and wrinkling, as well as our skin becoming thinner. Some women find their skin becomes itchier, too. Acne and increased facial hair growth can also occur during the menopause due to an imbalance of your hormones.

I always find it encouraging that our skin grows, replacing itself every few weeks from its base dermal layer, and it's to this that we need to pay the most attention and influence through what we put into our bodies. Applying enriched moisturising creams, serums formulated for more mature skins and richer body lotions are all likely to be soothing, comforting and a great morale booster, but a good skin starts with good nutrition, especially as we age.

Our skin and internal organs are supported by material called connective tissue, a cross between padding and scaffolding which holds everything in place. Under a microscope, this looks like weaving – thick and thin fibres of collagen and elastin mixed together, crisscrossing and forming an intricate mesh. Helping the skin in the continual process of renewal are the blood vessels, fat cells, hair follicles and nerve endings. Necessary to all this activity are hormones and oxygen, delivered to skin cells by the circulation of the blood. As early as our mid-thirties, this hormonal activity begins to slow up; the fat cells are reduced and the collagen and elastin become weaker, resulting in a number of negative visible effects on our skin (notably our faces).

The weakening of this support system and the reduction of its fat and moisture content causes the skin to wrinkle. The replacement of skin cells also slows down, so that the dead surface cells remain on the body for longer, becoming steadily drier through overexposure to the elements.

Starting from the foundation of our skin, as with many other aspects of health, a healthy diet is the basic necessity. Make sure that your body receives all the nutrients it needs and you may like to add in some optional extras to support the skin, such as collagen supplements and/or liquid hyaluronic acid (an internal skin moisturiser), as well as evening primrose oil (from the Rigel seed variety). Equally important is making sure that all nutrients are absorbed and utilised by the body effectively, which means keeping your blood circulation active – by exercising regularly.

Also, we have fewer melanocytes in our skin as we get older. These are the cells which contain the pigment melanin which is released to protect us against harmful UV rays when we're out in the sun. It's important to care for our skin from both the outside and the inside, though, and as there is a relationship between exposure to UV rays and skin cancer, it's vital that we wear a good sunscreen when outside in strong sunshine (especially on our face, neck and backs of the hands). Wearing a brimmed hat is a handy idea and lessens the need for so much sunscreen. I carry a cotton roll-up hat in my bag in case I get caught out by the vagaries of the Great British climate.

Any unusual skin changes such as a change in shape, size or pigmentation of a mole or the appearance of an unusual-looking mole should, of course, always be checked by your doctor or a specialist mole clinic (there are a number of these handy walk-in private screening centres now around the UK).

HAIR LOSS, GREYING AND HIRSUTISM

Oestrogen is very important for hair growth and when it decreases you may notice that your hair becomes thinner and less glossy. Some may find they brush out or find much more hair on their clothes than they are used to. This is normal, but unsettling. You may find yourself wanting a hairstyle that works well with thinner hair and may begin to realise why your mother has or had such a regular appointment at the hairdresser's. It may be worth considering having a liberating short crop and then letting nature run its course. Some women love their new shorter grey, greying or white hair, embracing their natural colour and the freedom from hair that needs blow-drying, styling and high maintenance. Of course, the reverse is also true and there are few easier or swifter ways to reverse the outward signs of ageing than covering grey hair with semi-permanent hair tints or soft blonde highlights woven between the grey (my own preferred method of disguise).

At around the same time, some women find that they get unwelcome thick and possibly dark hairs on their faces (so unfair to lose head hair while growing extra hair on the face!) particularly on the chin and above the upper lip. Keep a good pair of tweezers permanently in your bathroom and/or handbag to get rid of the hairs as soon as they appear (invest in a well-lit magnifying mirror). There are also more long-lasting solutions to this problem, including laser treatment, IPL (intense pulsed light), waxing, using depilatory cream, threading and electrolysis. If you're not keen on long dark hairs on your face and are long-sighted it's a good idea to make sure you inspect your face regularly when wearing your reading glasses to avoid a potentially 'Oh no!' situation when you return from a work or social gathering.

HEADACHES AND WORSENING MIGRAINES

You may experience headaches that occur more frequently as a result of your fluctuating hormone levels. These headaches can vary in intensity and be associated with nausea and vomiting. If you've had PMS-related migraines in the past, you may find that your migraines become more severe or closer together in their frequency. This can also be a sign that your hormone levels are changing.

Eating small amounts regularly – every three to four hours during the day – is a good way of preventing these headaches, as is making sure you get some regular 'me time' and drinking plenty of water – at least 1.5–2 litres daily, as headaches can often be a sign of simple dehydration. In addition, having the right dose and type of HRT can often really improve the frequency and severity of migraines.

VAGINAL DRYNESS AND URINARY SYMPTOMS

Vaginal dryness or atrophy, also called atrophic vaginitis, is a change to your vagina which develops when there is a significant decrease in oestrogen levels. Some doctors refer to it as a genitourinary syndrome of the menopause (GSM) as it's not just your vagina that is affected. Your urinary tract can also be affected by the low levels of oestrogen – and this can also lead to increased rates of urinary tract infections and cystitis. Vaginal dryness can also be caused by breastfeeding, taking the oral contraceptive pill, or some types of medications (such as anti-depressants, antihistamines or tamoxifen).

Oestrogen is important as a natural lubricant in your vagina and helps to keep this area healthy and moist. Oestrogen also stimulates the cells that line your vagina to produce glycogen. Glycogen is a compound which encourages the presence of helpful germs (bacteria) which protect your vagina from infections. This lack of oestrogen tends to cause the tissues around your vagina to become thinner, dryer and inflamed. These changes can take months or even years to develop and vary between women.

Your vagina may shrink a little and expand less easily during sex, making sexual intercourse more painful or uncomfortable (contributing to lowered libido). Your vulva (the external genitals: labia, clitoris and the entrance to the vagina) may become thin, dry and itchy. You may notice that your vulva or vagina has become red and sore. You may also find you have episodes of thrush more frequently. Many women have symptoms of vaginal pain and discomfort throughout the day, so it is often not just a problem to those women who are sexually active.

As the skin around your vagina becomes increasingly sensitive it is more likely to itch. This can make you prone to scratching, which in turn makes your skin more likely to itch, and so on. Using synthetic chemical products, such as medicated wipes, sprays, gels and antiseptics or even some types of washing powder (especially Biological), will almost certainly worsen vaginal dryness by altering the healthy balance of bacteria and pH levels and allowing unhealthy bacteria in to create infection (which causes itching, and so on).

It's really important to use gentle, non-scented soaps and pH-balanced washes for intimate cleaning; some women use only water and find this works very well. Eating a healthy diet that includes drinking plenty of water, eating fresh vegetables and taking probiotics such as plain, live yoghurt and kefir, and taking regular exercise helps good vaginal function – in particular walking and running help the pelvic floor to tone up, ensure good general health and help prevent constipation which can damage vaginal function. The stronger your pelvic floor, the less likely you are to accidentally pass urine (see pages 33–4).

In addition, the low levels of oestrogen in your body can lead to thinning and weakening of the tissues around the neck of your bladder, or around the opening for urine to pass (the urethra). For example, urinary symptoms that may occur include an urgency to get to the loo and recurring urinary infections or cystitis. Some women find that they cannot hold on to urine as effectively as they could before, which can even lead to episodes of urinary incontinence (see URINARY INCONTINENCE, pages 31–6).

All these symptoms can be present long after your menopause, even when you don't have any other symptoms. They are very common symptoms that affect the vast majority of women at some time after the menopause. You are also more likely to experience symptoms as more years pass after your menopause. They occur in at least 7 out of 10 women after the menopause and can occur even if you are taking hormone replacement therapy (HRT).

Many women don't seek help or advice from their doctor about vaginal dryness. This is very often because we're embarrassed and don't realise how common it is – or how its physical effects can impact on more than just our sex life. However, treating vaginal dryness can make a massive improvement to the quality of your life and it's helpful to seek help and appropriate treatment (see SOLUTIONS AND TREATMENTS FOR VAGINAL DRYNESS, pages 77–80).

– 7 –

Long-term Health Problems Arising From the Menopause

Although the menopause is a natural part of our life cycle, it causes physical changes that can negatively affect our health if they are not recognised and sorted out in good time.

OSTEOPOROSIS

Our bone tissue is made up of protein hardened by calcium salts and other minerals to make it strong. Bone tissue is alive and constantly changes throughout our life in order for it to be as healthy as possible. We have cells in our bodies that are constantly laying down new bone (osteoblasts) and other cells that are removing old bone (osteoclasts). Until we are around 25 years old, we normally build more bone than we lose. Past 30 years old, we can't build any more bone density and it becomes a matter of bone maintenance through our diet and exercise regime. However, during the menopause, bone breakdown happens at a faster rate than bone buildup, resulting in a loss of bone mass. Once this loss of bone reaches a certain point, that person has osteoporosis.

The drop in oestrogen levels during the menopause results in increased bone loss which leads to our bones becoming less dense and less strong. Around 10 per cent of a woman's bone mass is lost in the first five years of the menopause and this increases our risk of osteoporosis developing. At the age of 50, about one in 50 women have osteoporosis. This rises to one in four women at the age of 80. Men can also be affected and over a third of women and one in five men in the UK have one or more bone fractures because of osteoporosis in their lifetime. There are estimated to be 180,000 fractures every year in England and Wales caused by osteoporosis alone.

Those with osteoporosis have an increased risk of fracturing a bone – sometimes with little or no trauma involved, such as a fall. This means that normal activities such as sitting, standing, coughing or even hugging can on occasion result in painful fractures. These fractures can happen in any of our bones, including our spine, hips and wrists. This can cause us considerable pain and sometimes even disability.

It's very important to have good vitamin D levels because, as well as helping maintain a healthy immune system, this vitamin is important for keeping our bones healthy as it enables calcium (essential for healthy bones) to be absorbed. Vitamin D is made in the skin following sun exposure and is found in very small amounts in some foods, notably animal produce. To have adequate levels of vitamin D we need to be exposed to the midday sun for at least 20 minutes at least three times a week, every week (I do use a strong sunblock on my face, neck and backs of hands though). This is clearly not possible for most of us and has led to the government suggesting recently that we should all (in the UK) take vitamin D supplements in order to maintain healthy levels of this essential vitamin.

Again, it's vital to keep moving and exercising. Running, walking, yoga, tennis, golf, swimming, etc. are all fantastically good activities to keep us upbeat and healthy. They also help keep our bones strong and of course if you are running, swimming and walking outside, you'll automatically increase the amount of time you spend in the sun, synthesising essential and protective vitamin D through the skin.

Remember, though, if you have osteoporosis, no amount of exercise will help if you don't eat a healthy balanced diet; nutrients are as important as weight-bearing exercise. Not eating enough can be as damaging to your health as eating too much (see EATING DISORDERS AND THE MENOPAUSE, pages 96–7).

A healthy balanced diet, including foods rich in vitamin D, such as oily fish (think mackerel and salmon), cheese, egg yolks, beef liver and foods fortified with vitamin D (some cereals and dairy products and orange juice), will also help boost levels of this important vitamin.

CARDIOVASCULAR DISEASE

Cardiovascular disease means diseases of your heart and blood vessels, and they include heart attacks and strokes. Oestrogen is very important for keeping our blood vessels healthy as it seems to have a positive effect on the inner layer of the walls of our blood vessels. This helps to keep blood vessels flexible and healthy. Because levels of oestrogen decrease during the perimenopause, our risk of cardiovascular disease increases after the menopause.

Other changes in the cardiovascular system can take place, too. Your blood pressure is more likely to start to increase. In addition, bad cholesterol, or LDL cholesterol, levels may increase and those of good cholesterol, or HDL cholesterol, may decline or stay the same.

An increased risk of cardiovascular disease and also osteoporosis is far greater if you have an early menopause, especially if you have Premature Ovarian Insufficiency (POI). Your doctor will be able to discuss this with you in more detail and it's very helpful to know that this increased risk can be greatly reduced with hormone treatment.

To minimise your risk of cardiovascular disease, stop smoking, reduce your alcohol intake and keep exercising.

Eating a healthy balanced diet (see FOODS FOR HEALTH DURING AND AFTER THE MENOPAUSE, pages 90–7) with plenty of fresh fruit and vegetables, protein and complex carbohydrates (many of which are fruit and vegetables), wholewheat pasta and bread, brown rice and very little sugar will increase your energy levels, help make you feel fuller for longer and, for all the reasons above, will probably mean you will want to exercise more.

WEIGHT GAIN

Being overweight is known to increase the risk of getting many serious diseases, including some cancers and heart disease.

Oestrogen can affect both where we store fat in the body and also how it's burned. The menopause can cause our metabolism to slow, which can then contribute to weight gain. Many women notice that their body shape changes as they go through the menopause and they have more weight gain around their middle (literally, middle-age spread). This is something to be keenly aware of and avoid, as being overweight – especially round your middle – increases your risk of heart disease and some cancers.

Again, cut down on alcohol intake, keep exercising and eating a well-balanced diet with plenty of veggies and other plant-based foods (see FOODS FOR HEALTH DURING AND AFTER THE MENOPAUSE, pages 90–7), always with very little sugar. This will both help you maintain a healthy weight and increase your energy levels which, in turn, will make you more likely to carry on exercising . . .

A good, easy and healthy habit to adopt is drinking a large glass of water half an hour before every meal. Doing this means that: a) your stomach is not empty when you begin your meal, and b) we often mistake thirst for hunger so quenching your thirst before eating is a sensible way to eat only what you need. It's also a good way of keeping properly hydrated. When drinking wine, I also try to make sure I follow each glass of wine with a glass of water.

– 8 –

Managing your Menopause and the Importance of Friendship

It's important to be aware of the various medical treatments around that can work really well to improve your symptoms of the menopause and your health in general, including any potential benefits and risks, in order to make informed choices.

Talking about your symptoms to friends and your doctor is hopefully a really helpful way of dealing with them, by giving you the confidence to take action to improve your symptoms. Women are usually extremely supportive and happy to share their experiences and give advice, so keep talking! You'll probably be helping someone else while helping yourself. You'll also find that your symptoms are experienced by many more women than you might imagine, and, in my experience, this always makes a problem easier to deal with.

There is relatively new evidence to suggest that having friends and spending time with them can counteract the kind of stomach-churning stress many of us can experience on a daily basis. Research shows that women respond to stress with a cascade of brain chemicals that cause us to make, and maintain, friendships with other women. Until this study was published, most scientists believed that when under stress both sexes release hormones that enable the body to stand and fight, or flee (the fight or flight response). Now, some believe that women have a different response and that when oxytocin is released as part of the stress response, it buffers the fight or flight, response and encourages her to stay and look after her children and/or gather with other women instead. When she allows herself to engage in this tending or befriending, studies suggest that more oxytocin is released, which further counters stress and produces a calming effect. This calming response does not occur in men, because testosterone – which men produce in high levels when they're under stress – seems to reduce the effects of oxytocin. Oestrogen (our old friend!) on the other hand, appears to enhance it. Fascinating.

It may take some time for new studies to reveal all the ways in which oxytocin encourages us to care for children and spend time with other women, but the 'tend and befriend' notion developed by the researchers involved in this particular study may explain why women consistently outlive men. Study after study has found that social ties reduce our risk of disease by lowering blood pressure, heart rate and cholesterol. There's no doubt, they believe, that having friends is helping us live longer. It is also helping us live better.

A famous Harvard Medical School study (the Nurses' Health Study) found that the more friends women had, the less likely they were to develop physical impairments as they aged, and the more likely they were to be leading a joyful life. In fact, the results were so significant, the researchers concluded, that not having close friends or confidants was as detrimental to your health as smoking or carrying extra weight. So there is now an excuse to organise an outing with friends or to pick up the phone for a chat; it's really healthy!

We can see from this that there is every reason to make and maintain friendships but the truth is that often when we get very busy with work and family, the first thing we do is neglect these friendships. We might make our female friendships a low priority. This is a big mistake because women are such a source of strength to each other. We nurture one another and we need to make unpressured space and time in which we can do the special talk that women do when they're with other women. It's very healing and the menopause is a time — because it can coincide with other significant life pressures – when we really need our women friends close to us, to help us make wise decisions and choices that will ensure the rest of our life is as good as it can possibly be.

This is a moment to re-orientate your life; to make sure that every moment is positive and constructive. The first thing to do is to minimise any symptoms that have a negative influence on your life and explore every avenue of support. Then plans can be laid for the satisfying and exciting future that will almost certainly follow this interesting and natural time of change.

SCREENING PROGRAMMES

It's essential we keep up to date with cervical and breast screening programmes throughout our lives, even as we age and especially as our bodies begin to change through the menopause.

A cervical screening test (previously known as a smear test) is a crucial method of detecting abnormal cells on the cervix – the entrance to the womb from the vagina.

Detecting and removing abnormal cervical cells can prevent cervical cancer – the whole process is quick, simple and it works. Although cervical screening isn't a test for cancer itself, it does check the health of the cells of the cervix. The vast majority of test results show that everything is normal, but for around one in 20 women the test will show some abnormal changes in the cells of the cervix. Again, this shouldn't cause panic as most of these won't go on to lead to cervical cancer and the cells may go back to normal on their own, but in some cases the abnormal cells need to be removed so that they can't then become cancerous.

All women who are registered with a GP in England are invited for cervical screening. So if you're aged between 25 and 49 you can be screened every three years; if you're aged between 50 and 64 you can be screened every five years, and at over 65, only women who haven't been screened since the age of 50 or those who have recently had abnormal tests will be screened. In Scotland, screening starts at 20 years and continues three-yearly until the age of 60. You can also be screened on a self-pay basis, should you choose to do so, at privately funded GPs, well-women clinics and private hospitals.

Breast-screening aims to find breast cancers early. It uses an X-ray test called a mammogram that can spot cancers when they are too small to see or feel.

Breast-screening sometimes picks up cancers that may not have caused any symptoms or become life-threatening and you may end up having unnecessary extra tests and treatment. As the likelihood of getting breast cancer increases with age, all women who are between 50 and 70 years old (in many areas it is now 47 and 73 years) and registered with a GP are automatically invited for breast-cancer screening every three years. In the meantime, if you are worried about breast cancer symptoms, such as a lump or area of thickened tissue in a breast, don't wait to be offered screening – see your GP immediately. Again, self-pay mammograms are available privately.

HELPING THE SKIN

As our skin grows from its base dermal layer, replacing itself every few weeks, it's worth taking the time to focus on creating stronger, healthier-looking skin from within. The weakening of our skin's support system and the reduction of its fat and moisture content causes the skin to wrinkle. The replacement of skin cells also slows down, so that the dead surface cells remain on the body for longer, becoming steadily drier through overexposure to the elements. Starting from the foundation of our skin, as with so many areas of our health, a healthy diet is our daily, basic necessity. Make sure that your skin – and body – receives all the nutrients it needs. Equally important is making sure that these nutrients are absorbed and used by the body effectively and this means keeping our blood circulation active with movement and exercise.

We all have fewer melanocytes in our skin as we age. These are the cells which contain the protective pigment, melanin, released to protect our skin and insides against the harmful UV rays of the sun. With such a strong relationship between exposure to UV rays and skin cancer, it is vital that we wear a good sunscreen when the sun is at its strongest, or when spending lengthy periods of time outdoors. And, of course, any unusual signs of skin changes such as a change in shape, size or pigmentation of a mole should always be checked by a healthcare professional.

EXERCISE

Regular exercise obviously brings us many health benefits. Weight-bearing exercise that uses our body weight (such as jogging) and weight-resisted exercise (which involves pushing against some resistance, such as strength training) can both really help to improve the strength of our bones and we need to maintain a healthy weight to do this; being underweight is as unhealthy as being overweight. Trying to eat an appropriate amount of food that takes into account how much exercise you're taking makes you less likely to either over- or under-eat.

Regular exercise can reduce our risk of both osteoporosis and cardiovascular disease developing, and it's the best stress-buster around – along with time spent doing things that interest you and take you 'out of yourself'. Essentially, things that are completely absorbing and leave you unable to think about your everyday worries and concerns.

Walking for Health (see USEFUL CONTACTS, page 103) provides a countrywide network of groups of people to walk with. It's an excellent resource if you're single, newly widowed, have a husband or partner who doesn't like walking, or if you just don't have a dog and fancy getting out into the fresh air!

Recently the Spanish Menopause Society, the Spanish Cardiology Society and the Spanish Federation of Sports Medicine reviewed published studies on exercise during and after the menopause and interestingly found that while swimming, dancing and other forms of activity all have great benefits, Pilates, weight lifting and high-intensity interval training (HIIT) are likely to be the most beneficial.

A good Pilates class that will help you during this time should include lots of pulling/pushing movements, reaching, lifting and rotating, plus transitional movements like getting up and down from the floor. Flexibility and balance work are really good for preventing falls, and relaxation periods are valuable in helping to counteract any stress that exists during the often very busy perimenopausal phase of life. Another very important part of Pilates is the focus on the 'inner core' and strengthening our pelvic floor muscles. Totally invaluable. It's worth trying to find a menopause-friendly Pilates class; they're growing in popularity and there's nothing like demand to increase supply, so ask around your local area to see if one is available – or train and start one yourself!

High-intensity interval training (HIIT) involves doing short bursts of *very* hard exercise interspersed with rest periods and is particularly popular with time-pressed professionals, many of whom will be approaching or are in their perimenopause. So keep going! The researchers said that these forms of exercise are especially good because they improve balance, which in turn helps prevent falls. HIIT has also been shown to boost metabolism, so can also help prevent the onset of middle-age spread.

– 9 –

Hormone Replacement Therapy (HRT)

So – the elephant in the room is most often 'should I take HRT to help my menopausal symptoms?' You'll have noticed that the majority of the symptoms of the menopause are due to fluctuating and then low levels of the hormone oestrogen. All types of hormone replacement therapy (HRT) contain an oestrogen hormone, because HRT replaces the oestrogen that our ovaries either no longer make or supply in fluctuating levels during perimenopause. Women without a womb usually only need oestrogen (but some, according to symptoms, need testosterone too). A form of progestogen is given to those women with a womb and some may also need testosterone. The doses and types of hormones vary according to your medical history, symptoms and need and it's important to have a detailed discussion with your doctor and, if necessary, to get more specialised help with a GP who is expert in this area, or a private well-woman or menopause clinic. However, even low levels of basic HRT can be of significant benefit and improve your symptoms.

WHERE DOES HRT COME FROM?

The first form of hormone replacement therapy was created as long ago as 1890 and was called Ovarin, being quite literally made from bovine ovarian tissue. This was updated in the 1930s with the introduction of a product called Emminen, which was made from pregnant women's urine. As you might imagine, this was not that widely available, and as popularity grew, drug companies turned instead to pregnant mares to create Premarin, literally PREgnant MAres uRINe, extracting hormones from the urine of pregnant horses. This was essentially pure oestrogen, which later became linked with an increased risk of developing uterine (womb) cancer, and so a safer version called Prempak C was introduced, which combines conjugated horse oestrogens with a progestogen in one treatment. Today, these ingredients are very much less commonly used and most standard UK and European HRT formulations are plant-derived and come from the oestrogen-rich yam plant. Oestrogel and micronised progesterone, both commonly used in modern HRT, come from this tropical root vegetable. A substance called diosgenin, a precursor of progesterone, is also extracted from the yam plant and then undergoes several chemical reactions in order to become progesterone. This is absolutely identical to the hormone produced by the body.

It's always worth discussing your prescription, and its ingredients, with your doctor. If your GP doesn't know the answer s/he may refer you to an expert in the menopause if they feel they're not qualified to advise you properly. There are NHS menopause clinics you can ask to be referred to, offering very similar treatments to some pricey private clinics who so often charge a small fortune for their services. It's so much better to discuss any possible doubts about HRT as soon as possible – and try to resolve them – than to needlessly suffer symptoms that are adversely affecting your life.

Some private clinics offer what they call bio-identical hormones. However, some of these are very similar (if not identical) to most of those prescribed in the UK. The downside is that these are not regulated and are not subject to independent medical quality control, so make sure you do your research before you commit to anything – and check that any medication you take is NICE-approved (National Institute for Health and Care Excellence). NICE do not approve of bio-identical hormones and they are not licensed.

HRT is the most effective, clinically proven treatment available for relieving symptoms such as hot flushes, night sweats, joint pains, mood swings and urinary symptoms. And for the vast majority of us under 60 years old, the benefits of HRT outweigh the risks. HRT is also recommended for young women if they have an early menopause; they will need to take it until they are at least 51 years old.

However, it's easy to feel confused about the different types of HRT available as well as about the benefits and risks of taking it. It's important that your own individual health is taken into consideration by your doctor when discussing HRT. Some women may choose not to take HRT or others may not be able to take HRT due to an underlying medical condition. If you're not sure whether or not it is appropriate for you, do discuss this with your doctor. If the answer is no – for whatever reason – it may be worth seeking a second opinion from a specialist.

There is no set length of time that you should take HRT for; some women take it for a few years, others for longer. (See HOW LONG CAN YOU TAKE HRT FOR?, pages 75–6) It's usually an individual decision taken after discussion between you and your doctor.

Be warned, though, that HRT does not work as a contraceptive. So if you need contraception, do talk to your doctor about the best options available to you. See CONTRACEPTION FOR THE OVER 40s, pages 15–18, for more information.

TYPES OF HRT

HRT is available as tablets, skin patches or gel – or even as a combination of these. The skin patches and gel are absorbed through the skin and may be considered preferable to tablets, which need to be processed via the liver. Normally, it's extremely hard for anything to get through the skin, so these two kinds of treatment are unusual in this respect. The patches, such as Elleste Solo or Evorel, work by placing an occlusive sticking plaster-like barrier over the skin. This keeps the hormone loaded onto the patch in direct contact with the skin 24/7. The patches are usually changed twice a week. The oestrogen gel, such as Oestrogel, is made with the emulsifier triethanolamine, which is unusually compatible with both lipids (oils) and water, making it more easily absorbed into the body through the epidermis (outer layer of skin). One or two pumps from the pack are usually applied each day or night. Tablets are relatively straightforward to take and it's often handier to take the progesterone tablets, such as Utrogestan, last thing at night as they can make you feel slightly sleepy (a helpful side effect at bedtime).

If you still have a womb (uterus) you'll be given progestogen to take with the oestrogen. This is an essential part of the combination as taking oestrogen can cause the lining of the womb to build up, which can then increase your risk of cancer. However, taking a progestogen completely reverses this risk. This means that there is no increased risk of cancer of your womb if you take HRT.

If you're still having regular periods, then you'll be given a type of HRT that gives you a monthly period. This type of HRT needs to be taken for around a year. If you haven't had a period for one year, or if you have taken HRT for one year, then it's likely you'll be given a type of HRT which does not give you a period. It can be common and completely normal to have some light bleeding or spotting in the first few months of using this type of HRT. However, if you experience heavy or prolonged vaginal bleeding do talk to your doctor.

If you have a history of a clot, migraine, diabetes or liver disease you can still take HRT but it is likely that you'll be recommended to use a patch or gel rather than a tablet. This is safer and associated with less risks compared to having the tablet form of oestrogen. The progestogen is usually still given as a tablet, though. The hormones given are usually body-identical, which means that they are the same composition as the hormones that your body produces.

If you and your doctor decide your symptoms warrant taking HRT, you may want to ask for 17 beta oestradial, which is pure oestrogen and more commonly used nowadays. It has the same molecular structure as the oestrogen that our bodies produce. You may also want to ask for micronised progesterone, which is body-identical and less likely to cause unwanted side effects than progestogens.

There are numerous different preparations and doses of HRT and if one type does not suit you, it's very likely that another one will.

BENEFITS

Many women wait until their symptoms are really troublesome or even unbearable before starting HRT. However, taking HRT early really will make a difference to your symptoms (and quality of life) and also lead to a greater improvement in your heart and bone health. There is no advantage in waiting until your symptoms become really bad or even unbearable before starting on HRT.

Many women find that all their menopause symptoms improve within a few months of taking HRT and feel that they have their 'old life' and their 'old self' back again. They often notice that both their sleep and mood improve and their concentration recovers, too. They also often discover that their energy is much greater than it was before they started taking HRT. They may just feel happier in themselves.

HRT usually works to stop hot flushes and night sweats within a few weeks. In addition, HRT will reverse many of the changes around your vagina and vulva, usually within one to three months. However, it can take up to a year of treatment in some cases. This means that HRT can improve symptoms of vaginal dryness, improve discomfort during intercourse, help to reduce recurrent urine infections and also improve any increased frequency of passing urine. You may still need some other treatment for vaginal dryness, though (see pages 77–80). You may find that any aches or pains in your joints improve, as does the texture of your hair and skin, when taking HRT.

If you're still experiencing menopausal symptoms on HRT then your dosage will probably be increased. Alternatively, changing the formulation of HRT can make a difference – for example, changing from taking a tablet to using a patch.

There is some evidence that taking HRT, especially HRT with oestrogen alone, actually reduces our risk of developing cardiovascular disease (heart attacks especially) in women. The benefits are greatest in those women who start HRT within 10 years of their menopause.

HRT can also lower cholesterol levels, and this is beneficial for our heart and body overall. Taking HRT does not increase your risk of heart disease if you start taking it when you are under 60 years old. In addition, it does not affect your risk of dying from heart disease. Certainly, up until the age of 60, the benefits of taking HRT usually outweigh the risks.

Oestrogen also helps to keep our bones strong and healthy. Taking HRT, even if we are only take low doses of it, can prevent and reverse the bone loss that occurs. This means that taking HRT reduces our risk of osteoporosis and also of having a fracture due to osteoporosis. This benefit is maintained during treatment but does reduce when we stop taking HRT. However, there is some evidence that this reduction in risk of fracture persists for a time even after HRT is stopped.

Some studies have shown a reduced risk of Alzheimer's disease and other types of dementia in women who take HRT. However, other studies have not shown this, so more work needs to be done in this area. In addition, some studies have also shown a reduction in risk of bowel cancer in women who take HRT. However, again, the evidence for this is still not completely clear.

According to Professor John Studd, consultant gynaecologist, senior lecturer and a pioneer of the combined oestrogen/progesterone treatment, there are 10 good reasons to be happy about HRT:

- It stops hot flushes and sweats

- It treats vaginal dryness

- It increases bone density and prevents osteoporotic fractures

- It protects intervertebral discs, reducing 'dowager's hump'

- It reduces the incidence of heart attacks

- It helps the symptoms of depression in many women

- It improves libido

- It improves the texture of the skin

- It improves mood and reduces irritability

- It is safe.

TESTOSTERONE

Testosterone is the third hormone that can work alongside oestrogen and progesterone when talking about HRT. Our normal levels dramatically reduce during the menopause as our ovaries stop working, which can be an issue as testosterone helps boost our mood, energy levels, concentration and sex drive (libido). Low levels in our body are usually diagnosed by two blood tests; one for basic testosterone levels and another called SHBG (sex hormone binding globulin), which assesses total bio-available testosterone. When levels of testosterone reduce, we desire sex less often than we used to and sex may not be as pleasurable as it used to be, even though you still fancy your partner. Taking testosterone can help reverse this.

It's a highly personal choice. One GP I spoke to on this subject said some women ask her for testosterone to help boost their sex drive, only to often come off it after six months or so. On the other hand, I have also spoken to women who swear by it for resurrecting their middle-aged love life! Some women also find taking testosterone improves clarity of thinking, with one reporting that after just a few months of testosterone supplements her brain-fog had lifted and overall her thinking was 'far crisper'. This is logical when you consider that we have so much testosterone circulating around our system naturally in our early years. Testosterone is usually given as a topical skin gel or sometimes as an implant. The dose of testosterone is very low so it won't cause facial hair growth or a deeper voice . . . and it's usually prescribed by a doctor who specialises in the menopause. It is available on the NHS, but most often only from specialist GPs or menopause clinics. If you think you might benefit, do ask your GP for a referral.

HRT RISKS

Many women are scared or worried about HRT because of the potential risks of taking it. There is no question that there's been a huge amount of media attention on this subject, in particular after the results of some large studies about HRT were published over a decade ago. These studies raised concerns over the safety of HRT, primarily over a possible increased risk of breast cancer with HRT and also a possible increased risk of heart disease. However, the reporting of these studies have since been shown to be inaccurate and flawed. In recent years there have been other studies which have shown how safe HRT is, and that although it can increase your risk of developing certain problems, this increase is very small in most cases.

Your actual risk from taking HRT depends on many factors (such as whether you smoke, your weight, your age, family history of certain conditions and also your general health), so it's not just whether or not you take HRT that affects your risks. This is why it is very important for you and your doctor to discuss the risks and benefits to you as an individual of taking HRT.

Breast cancer is still the risk that most women worry about with HRT. It is true that you may have a small increased risk of breast cancer if you take HRT containing oestrogen and a progestogen. However, if you are taking oestrogen-only HRT then you actually have a lower risk of breast cancer compared to a woman who is not taking HRT.

The risk associated with taking the combined HRT does increase the longer you use HRT, but when you stop taking it, you have the same risk of breast cancer as someone who has not taken the treatment. So the increased risk of breast cancer in this situation is very small – in fact, similar to the increased risk of breast cancer in women who are obese, those women who have never had children and also those women who drink two to three units of alcohol each day. There has never been a study that has indisputably shown there is an increased risk of dying from breast cancer in women who take HRT.

The findings of a study published in the *British Journal of Cancer* in August 2016 suggested that the increased risk of breast cancer among women taking the more common combined HRT in the longer term is slightly higher than previous studies have shown; their results showed closer to a threefold increase rather than a doubling for those taking HRT for over 15 years. However, according to British GP and menopause expert, Dr Louise Newson, there is no new cause for alarm. 'The results of this study are similar with other studies in that women who are only taking oestrogen (i.e. those women who have had a hysterectomy) do not have an increased risk of breast cancer. It appears to be the type of progestogen that is important and the newer type of progestogen, micronised progesterone, and also the Mirena coil, were not mentioned in this study. It is very important for women to understand that there are so many other risk factors for breast cancer. These include being overweight or obese, being older, drinking alcohol and smoking. The risk of developing breast cancer is actually greater if you are overweight than if you take HRT. Any increased risk of breast cancer with taking HRT is reversed on stopping HRT.'

Most of the studies that look at the association of breast cancer and HRT have not shown an increased risk of breast cancer in women who take HRT for five years or less. Women who take combined HRT have an increased risk of having an abnormal mammogram, as HRT can increase the density of your breast tissue. This is not the same as increasing the risk of breast cancer.

Note: There is *no* increased risk of breast cancer in women who take HRT under the age of 51 years.

Women who take HRT as tablets have a small increased risk of developing a blood clot. You're more likely to develop a clot if you're obese, have had a clot in the past or are a smoker. However, there's no increased risk of developing a blood clot if you use oestrogen patches or gel, rather than tablets of HRT.

Some studies have shown that there is a small increased risk of stroke in women taking either oestrogen-only or the combined HRT. But again, there's no increased risk of this in women who use oestrogen patches or gel rather than the tablets. In addition, oral HRT containing lower doses of oestrogen seems to be associated with a lower risk of stroke compared to those containing higher doses. Most women under the age of 60 years have a very low risk of stroke.

SIDE EFFECTS OF HRT

Side effects are more likely to occur when you first start taking HRT and they usually settle with time. The most common side effects in the first few weeks are a feeling of sickness (nausea), some breast discomfort and possibly leg cramps. But these are all relatively rare.

HOW LONG CAN YOU TAKE HRT FOR?

There's no one answer to this question, and the length of time for which a woman takes HRT is variable. Some women take it for a few years to help improve their worst symptoms of the menopause. After this, many find they then have no more symptoms of the menopause. If your symptoms return when you stop taking HRT, this isn't an effect of taking hormones, but because you'd still be having symptoms of the menopause anyway. HRT doesn't delay the menopause, it simply masks the symptoms while you're going through it. It's a daily treatment with no accumulative effect – as soon as you stop, your body reverts to its natural hormone level at that moment in time, with no ongoing benefits.

Some women decide to take HRT for much longer than a few years. This is often because they feel better and have more energy when taking it – and also because they know they will benefit from a reduced risk of osteoporosis and heart disease. How long you take it for really is an individual decision between yourself and your doctor, and is usually reviewed on an annual basis. From 60 years of age onwards, you may simply need to adjust the dosage and keep taking HRT for its benefits of increased bone density, heart disease protection, as well as the improved condition of hair, skin and nails. It's a matter of personal choice.

– 10 –

Solutions and Treatments for Vaginal Dryness

Probably the least discussed symptom of the menopause is vaginal dryness. It's not a topic that many of us find easy to discuss but, for so many reasons, it is worth talking about – not least because the solution is usually very easily found and the ramifications of not finding a solution can be so negative; a less than satisfying and probably dwindling sex life and an increased risk of UTIs (urinary tract infections).

For those who address the problem, the rewards are great; a more satisfying sex life and the knowledge that you're helping to protect yourself against urinary tract infections (regardless of whether you're having sex or not).

This condition can usually be treated very easily. As the problem is usually due to lack of oestrogen, the usual treatment is replacing the oestrogen in your vagina and the surrounding tissues. A cream, vaginal tablet or ring containing oestrogen is often prescribed and they all work really well. A vaginal tablet is a very small tablet that you insert into your vagina with a small applicator. The vaginal tablets and creams are usually used every day for two weeks, and then used twice a week thereafter. The ring is a soft, flexible ring with a centre that contains the oestrogen hormone and releases a steady, low dose of it each day over three months.

Using topical, targeted oestrogen in this way is not the same as taking hormone replacement therapy (HRT) and therefore doesn't have the same – usually very small – risks associated with it. This is because these preparations work to restore oestrogen 'down below' without giving oestrogen to your whole body. Of course, the downside of this is that topical oestrogen won't help any of the other menopausal symptoms you may suffer, such as night sweats and aching joints. However, these topical preparations can be safely used by most women and can also be used on a regular basis over a long period of time (usually indefinitely) as your symptoms will usually return if you stop this treatment.

Vaginal lubricants and moisturisers can be used either with hormones or on their own and are usually very effective. They're available either from your doctor on prescription, or to buy off the shelf from chemists. There are many different products available so there is plenty of choice to find one that suits you.

The alternative to applying a lubricant every time you have sex is to use an oestrogen-based treatment that you only have to apply a couple of times a week. Some products are sold with an applicator to enable discreet use and it's this sort of thing that's worth considering before you choose your method. Moisturisers are used regularly, whereas lubricants are solely used during intercourse. YES has a range of Certified Organic Products including a water-based intimate moisturiser/lubricant. Sylk is also a natural water-based intimate moisturiser which can also be used as lubricant. Both Sylk and YES water-based products are available on prescription and can be bought online or over the counter.

Many women use a combination of topical oestrogen and moisturisers/lubricants, and this is very effective and safe. Whichever method you decide on to treat vaginal dryness, the upside is that, very often, a rather predictable sex life established during years or even decades of marriage is likely to be reinvigorated as a result. If the successful treatment coincides with fewer dependents living at home, or a lessening of work hours or retirement, so much the better. Good sex is a good way of releasing tension and reconnecting with your other half.

It's important to find a formulation here that is free from potential skin irritants. Some lubricants may cause irritation, especially the 'stimulating' variety. The pH of the lubricant is also important – if it's too alkaline it can lead to urinary tract infections or thrush occurring. You should check on the packet for a product that is pH balanced, ideally between pH3.8 and pH4.5. Oil-based lubricants are not suitable for use with condoms, but otherwise are fine.

If you find a product irritates, stop using it and try another variety, as the ingredients in each product can be very different. Some women use K-Y jelly, but although this is what some doctors use for internal examinations, it's not an effective lubricant for vaginal dryness. Taking HRT systemically (tablets, gel or patches) can also improve these symptoms. However, some women who take HRT need these local treatments in addition and it's completely safe to use vaginal oestrogen together with HRT.

Your symptoms should improve after about three months of treatment with topical oestrogen. Do see your doctor if your symptoms don't improve, as sometimes they can be due to other conditions. It is also very important to see your doctor if you have any unusual bleeding if you're on any kind of hormone treatment. For more information on products that will help in this area see USEFUL CONTACTS, page 102.

– 11 –

Alternative Treatments and Helpful Strategies

There are some alternative medications that your doctor can prescribe for some of your symptoms. Some types of anti-depressants, such as citalopram or venlafaxine, can improve hot flushes in some women – even those who are not depressed. These medications are often not given for this reason, though. Other medications can sometimes be given and help some women, but their use is often limited by side effects (such as nausea or worsening libido).

Some women consider taking complementary and/ or alternative treatments to HRT for their menopause symptoms. There is a huge market of options available and products include red clover, black cohosh and St John's wort. However, many have limited clinical research and some are associated with significant risks to your health, especially if you are not being professionally advised or you fail to notice which products should not be taken in conjunction with others. These remedies are not currently recommended by the NHS for their use for the treatment of menopausal symptoms, so your doctor is unlikely to be clued up on the latest herbal or dietary remedy. However, many women do find them helpful, and if your symptoms are very mild and you do your research properly, they may help – particularly if you use a qualified herbalist to help you decide whether you can be helped and by what. See USEFUL CONTACTS, page 102, for further information.

The following are some of the most recommended and available herbal blends over the counter:

HERBAL REMEDIES

Agnus castus (*Vitex agnus-castus*)

This herb is reputed to work on the pituitary gland, which sends the message down to the ovary to release hormones. Agnus castus is potentially helpful as a hormone modulator in perimenopausal years and herbalists tend to use this herb as a first course of treatment for early onset of symptoms, including mood swings, tension and anxiety.

Black cohosh (*Cimicifuga racemosa*)

Usually the herb most recommended for relief of hot flushes and night sweats. There has been some evidence that this herb works as a SERM (selective oestrogen receptor modulator) despite a few very rare cases of liver damage (which may or may not have been linked to taking the herb). The National Institutes of Health in the US publishes updated safety information on this (and other) herbal treatments and this is worth reading before deciding when and what to take. It's not clear that the benefits of taking black cohosh are significantly more than the benefits that would be expected from taking a placebo (dummy pill).

Dong quai (*Angelica sinensis*)

This traditional Chinese medical herb is a mainstay of TCM (traditional Chinese medicine) and may be helpful for both hot flushes and night sweats. Herbalists may use dong quai for disturbed sleep and settling hormone-related insomnia.

Flax (*Linum usitatissimum*)

A plant grown for food and fibre, the seeds of flax plants come from the pretty blue flowers that are increasingly seen growing in farmers' fields. The seeds are known as either linseeds or flaxseeds and are a good source of essential fatty acids, notably omega-3 (keep fresh linseeds in a cool, dark place or in the fridge to prevent rancidity). Linseeds are also rich in phytoestrogens, so called as they are plant-derived (from the Latin *phyto*) with oestrogen-like activity. These include isoflavonoids, including lignan, also found in sesame. Lignan is important to help feed the beneficial bacteria in our gut, specifically those responsible for converting isoflavonoids into compounds with oestrogenic activity. But for best effect, we do need to boost our overall beneficial gut bacteria to support this process, which is killed off with a poor diet and medications such as antibiotics.

Kwao krua (*Pueraria mirifica*)

Coming from Thailand, the dry, powdered roots of this Asian plant have long been used in traditional folk medicine as a tonic, especially for women, and it is now officially regulated by the government agencies that control traditional Thai medicine. Its name comes from the Latin *puer* 'child' and *mirificus* 'miraculous'. Kwao krua is showing some promise as a herbal treatment for symptoms of the menopause and has been found to be a rich source of plant phytoestrogens. However, it has also been shown to have cytotoxic (cell-killing) properties and should only be taken under professional guidance.

Red clover (*Trifolium pratense*)

A legume plant in the same family as peanuts and beans, red clover has been shown to be rich in phytoestrogens that can help reduce the severity of menopausal symptoms, notably hot flushes and vaginal dryness. Researchers at the University of Maryland Medical Center have found red clover to be especially helpful for mimicking the effects of oestrogen, improving blood circulation, maintaining bone mineral density and even lowering inflammation of the skin. The phytoestrogens in red clover include isoflavones, coumestrol and flavonoids, and it is the isoflavones that can act like oestrogen within the body. Red clover can be taken in capsules, tincture or dried herbs used to make a tea. One of the most popular and potentially effective herbal remedies for menopausal symptoms.

Soya bean (*Glycine max*)

Like the flax plant, soya beans are rich in isoflavones and have been well documented as having beneficial phytoestrogen activity. Soya beans are legumes, like peanuts and beans, classified as an oilseed product in the US as they contain such a high amount of high-protein oil. Made into many food products, soya beans are processed into low-cost, high-protein foods, including textured vegetable protein (TVP) used in processed foods, as well as dairy substitutes such as soya milk. Soya beans are the mainstay of many Japanese and Asian foods, from traditional soya milk and tofu to fermented soya foods such as soy sauce, miso and tempeh. Oriental women who eat these foods every day have been shown to have far fewer menopausal symptoms, such as hot flushes and vaginal dryness. Soya is the most widely genetically modified crop in the world. If you're looking for non-GM soya, always check the pack for details or choose organic soya, which is always non-GM in origin.

Star anise (*Illicium verum*)

This star-shaped dried spice has an aniseed flavour (hence its name) and comes from a small evergreen tree in southwest China. Its distinctive flavour gives sambuca, Galliano and pastis liqueurs their unique taste. It has many interesting medicinal properties, being anti-bacterial, anti-fungal and a useful expectorant for coughs. How it may benefit menopausal symptoms is less clear, but it is probably due to its phytoestrogenic compounds diantheole and photoantheole. Traditionally used by some medical herbalists for female disorders, including PMS and low libido.

HERBAL SAFETY

To help keep herbal remedies safe, the UK regulatory bodies have developed a system called Traditional Herbal Registration (THR). Any herbal products that have been approved by this system have a THR logo on their packs, so if you're thinking about exploring the use of herbs for your symptoms, look out for products with this on. Herbal (or natural) products do not necessarily mean safe products. Keep in mind that although helpful for some, herbal remedies are not regulated by a medicine authority and they should not be considered simply a safer alternative to HRT, as there is so much variety in their effectiveness and potency. Many herbal medicines have unpredictable doses and purity. In addition, some products have significant side effects and can interfere with other medicines. These include liquorice, St John's wort, ginseng and even grapefruit.

Although some natural remedies may help with some symptoms of the menopause, they don't sort out the principle issue of low levels of hormones, so these plants will not necessarily improve the strength of our bones or reduce our risk of cardiovascular disease.

On the plus side, though, many women feel that some herbs do relieve their menopausal symptoms and, of course, if the symptoms are alleviated, a better night's sleep and a feeling of wellbeing is more likely. Even something as simple as a cup of chamomile or valerian tea last thing at night will encourage a better night's sleep and many women find that lemon balm tea and red clover flowers tea helpful with the insomnia brought on by night sweats.

AROMATHERAPY

Essential oils are fragrant, volatile oils produced from different parts of aromatic plants. They're highly concentrated and are generally best used diluted and blended in carrier oils before coming into contact with skin. The smell or inhalation of these highly fragrant essences can help shift mood or uplift the senses by a swift and direct effect on the limbic system within the brain (the area responsible for feelings and emotion). Essential oils can be used in the bath or for massage which is, of course, a wonderful way of relaxing, too. The following are most commonly used by aromatherapists, with their potential uses:

- Bergamot may help reduce depression
- Clary sage may be useful for PMS
- Fennel may help alleviate water retention
- Geranium may help with anxiety and feelings of restlessness
- Jasmine may help with depression, tension and anxiety
- Juniper may have a detoxifying effect
- Lavender may be useful in aiding sleep
- Rosemary may help prevent fluid retention when used regularly for massage.

There are many others, but all essential oils are often best recommended by an experienced therapist. The whole feeling is most enjoyable when combined with a good massage technique.

Although little has been proven about the effect of aromatherapy specifically on menopausal symptoms, any therapy which allows you valuable 'time out' is an investment in yourself and will help you cope better with menopause symptoms.

RELAXATION

A few simple relaxation techniques – turning off your television, phone and computer is as good a start as any – will help minimise your symptoms and encourage a good night's sleep. Yoga, acupuncture, cranial osteopathy, aromatherapy, reflexology, meditation and shiatsu are all likely to relax you and help you feel good. Some will also help with your fitness and energy levels and may help you avoid the toxic cycle of sleeplessness and tiredness that you might be in. You may try to counteract this (tiredness) cycle with caffeine and alcohol, which are, of course, the very things that will increase the severity and frequency of, or worsen, any hot flushes and sleeplessness you may experience.

– 12 –

Foods for Health During and After the Menopause

As I've mentioned before, eating a healthy balanced diet is so very important for everyone at any stage of their life, but especially so during the menopause. Eating well now will help you maintain the energy you need in your busy mid-life and stand you in good stead later, bolstering your armour against both osteoporosis and heart disease – two of the diseases that may strike either during or after your menopause. The foods that will decrease your risk of developing heart disease, diabetes, osteoporosis and cancer at this time of life include unrefined and unprocessed 'whole' grains (such as brown rice instead of white rice), plenty of green and colourful veggies and some fruit. To decrease the bone loss that's likely due to lower levels of oestrogen, pay very special attention to the two main nutrients associated with bone health and get plenty of them; calcium and vitamin D.

Good sources of calcium are dairy products, egg yolks,

bread (mostly fortified with calcium in their enriched baking flours), some green leafy vegetables including cabbage, broccoli and kale, pulses (lentils, chickpeas, peas; most beans, e.g. butter, runner, broad, haricot, cannellini, kidney, etc., including baked beans – which are actually haricot beans), nuts, dried fruit and fish that's eaten with bones, e.g. small fish such as whitebait or tinned sardines.

Spinach has a high calcium content but contains substances called oxalates which bind the calcium and prevent it being absorbed. Some mineral waters and foods with added calcium can also provide considerable amounts of calcium, so if you replace dairy milk with soya milk, look out for products that are enriched with this essential nutrient. Also, many other everyday foods, such as juices or breakfast cereals, contain added calcium.

Very high intakes of vitamin A may have a negative effect on your bones and make them more likely to fracture when you're older. If you regularly eat liver and liver products, avoid taking supplements containing more than 1.5mg of vitamin A per day. Stick to the recommended daily doses given on the packs of fish liver oil supplements, such as cod liver oil, as these are often high in vitamin A.

THE IMPORTANCE OF VITAMIN D

Vitamin D is very important for calcium absorption and a healthy immune system. Important vitamin D sources are oily fish, eggs, red meat (better to eat high-quality, locally reared, grass-fed red meat occasionally than to eat cheaper red meat more often) and foods voluntarily fortified with vitamin D by the manufacturer, such as some breakfast cereals and dairy products. However, it is difficult to obtain the levels of vitamin D that we need with food alone. This is due to the fact we also need to spend time in the sun to make vitamin D and the amount of time most of us spend outside in the summer sun (without necessarily being covered in sun protection products or wearing a hat and long sleeves) has decreased significantly. For this reason, the government has recently issued advice that says most of us (in the UK) should take vitamin D supplements during the winter months – 10mcg per day is enough for most of us, but it's worth discussing this with your doctor, particularly if you or they think you may be at risk of osteoporosis.

EAT RIGHT TO FEEL BRIGHT

Here are a few food tips to help keep us happier and healthier during and after the menopause:

- Avoid snacking on sugary foods – a sharp rise in your blood glucose level may be followed by a dip, which leaves you feeling tired and drained. Nuts and fresh fruit will restore your energy levels in a more balanced way and help keep energy levels stable.

❄ We need fewer calories as we get older, so drinking a glass of water before eating a meal, reducing your refined sugar intake and eating wholemeal flour and pasta, brown rice and porridge all help to keep us feeling fuller for longer and less likely to reach for sugary snacks.

❄ Stop eating foods likely to trigger or worsen hot flushes and night sweats, including stimulants such as coffee, alcohol, spicy foods and high cocoa-percentage chocolate – especially during the late afternoon or at night.

❄ Red Rooibos (redbush) tea is rich in trace elements and minerals, including iron, calcium, potassium, copper, manganese, zinc and magnesium. It's also completely caffeine-free. In South Africa, where most of it is grown, it's drunk with a dash of milk and sometimes a taste of honey.

❄ Seeds (sunflower, almonds and pumpkin) and legumes (peanuts, peas and beans) contain vitamin E, zinc and calcium. These nutrients and the oils in nuts and seeds work towards preventing dry skin and help normalise hormone levels.

❄ Protein foods which contain tryptophan (found in turkey, cottage cheese, oats and legumes) help manufacture the neurotransmitter serotonin in the brain, helping to control sleep and appetite and feeling upbeat.

❧ Eat more alkaline foods – vegetables, fruits, seeds, nuts and plain, live yoghurt; they help prevent calcium loss from your bones.

❧ Eat foods rich in magnesium and boron, minerals which are important for the replacement of bone and help reduce risk of osteoporosis; apples, pears, grapes, dates, raisins, legumes and nuts are good sources of boron.

❧ Phytoestrogens found in certain foods are compounds that can bind with oestrogen receptor sites in the body's cells, increasing the oestrogenic effect. By acting in a similar way to oestrogen, they may help to keep hormones a little more balanced. Soya milk and flour, linseeds, tofu, tempeh and miso, pumpkin seeds, sesame seeds, sunflower seeds, celery, rhubarb and green beans all contain phytoestrogens.

MENOPAUSE CAKE

Packed with phytoestrogens, the naturally occurring oestrogen-like compounds found in soya, linseeds and some dried fruits, this cake is not going to sort out all your menopausal needs, but it makes a nice end to this little book and a mug of tea and slice of cake is a bit of fun to break the ice when talking about your symptoms (or those of family and friends). Made with soya flour, soya milk and linseeds, it's wonderfully rich and moist, with a dense texture and a good, rich flavour. Just one slice is incredibly filling and can be used as a meal substitute in its own right. Store in an airtight tin or slice and freeze to eat as required. It is delicious, so do try it – and enjoy!

INGREDIENTS

100g linseeds*

100g spelt flour (or wholemeal wheat flour)

100g medium rolled oats

100g soya flour

100g raisins

200g pitted dates, chopped

100g dried apricots, chopped

50g sunflower seeds

50g sesame seeds, lightly toasted

50g flaked almonds, lightly toasted

2 tsp ground ginger

2 tsp ground cinnamon

4–5 pieces of stem ginger in syrup, chopped

500–600ml soya milk

2 tbsp honey

* linseeds are the same as flaxseeds

Note: it's important to use soya milk here for its phytoestrogens

METHOD

1. Whizz the linseeds in a food processor to crack open the shells, then place all the dry ingredients into a large bowl, along with the chopped stem ginger. Stir in 500ml of the soya milk and the honey and stir until the mixture has fully combined. Leave to soak for 30 minutes.

2. Preheat the oven to 190°C/375°F/Gas mark 5. Line a small loaf or round cake tin with baking parchment. Add the remaining 100ml of soya milk to the mixture to loosen, if needed, and spoon the mixture into the tin (it should drop easily from the spoon – add a little more soya milk if the mixture seems too dry or dense). Bake for about 1 hour or until a sharp knife comes out of the centre cleanly. Turn out onto a wire rack and leave to completely cool before slicing with a very sharp knife.

EATING DISORDERS AND THE MENOPAUSE

Eating disorders are increasingly common among menopausal women and some find that their menopause symptoms lead to the recurrence of an eating disorder that has been successfully managed in the past. The physical effects of an eating disorder are often more severe for a middle-aged woman than for a teenager. This is because weight loss associated with an eating disorder can lead to lower levels of oestrogen in someone whose levels are already low. In addition, if a woman is starving or purging her food, malnutrition and higher levels of the stress hormone cortisol can result in enormous bone loss, at a higher rate than occurs naturally during the menopause. Clearly, this also increases the risk of developing osteoporosis, with all the potential complications this may lead to.

It is really important to recognise that, with the right help, eating disorders can be effectively managed and women can recover. If you think you are newly suffering from an eating disorder or suspect the recurrence of one that you have successfully managed in the past, do see your GP for advice and a referral where appropriate. Left untreated, you risk significant damage to your bones, gut and immune system.

See USEFUL CONTACTS, page 103, for links to organisations that can help you manage an eating disorder.

GLOSSARY

Acupuncture – a traditional Chinese system of healing that involves the use of thin metal needles which are inserted into specific points beneath the skin to relieve symptoms.

Aromatherapy – the therapeutic use of herbal essential oils to treat many kinds of disorders, including hormonal problems, skin complaints and stress.

Climacteric – the medical name for the three stages of the menopause.

Cranial osteopathy – a gentle treatment working on the bones and fascia around the skull (cranium). Cranial osteopaths are much more highly trained than craniosacral therapists.

Herbalism – a natural form of medicine which uses various parts of plants to relieve certain conditions.

HIIT (high intensity interval training) – short bursts of hard exercise interspersed with rest periods.

HRT – hormone replacement therapy.

Oestrogen – oestrogen is three different hormones (oestradiol, oestrone and oestriol) that are produced by your body. Oestrogen has over 300 functions in maintaining the health of your skin, muscles, hair, digestion and brain. Used in HRT.

Osteoporosis – a degenerative disease caused by thinning of the bones and a loss of bone mass over time.

Pilates – Pilates, or the Physical Mind method, is a series of non-impact exercises designed by Joseph Pilates to develop strength, flexibility, balance and inner awareness.

Progesterone – another of the female hormones, this is the principal hormone secreted by the ovary as part of the menstrual cycle that prepares the uterus to receive and sustain fertilised eggs. Also used in HRT.

Progestogen – progestogens are synthetic forms of progesterone. Used in HRT.

Reflexology – a form of therapeutic foot massage which is used to relieve pain and tension by stimulating predefined pressure points on the feet and hands. Sometimes used in conjunction with aromatherapy. It should not be used as an alternative to seeking medical advice.

Shiatsu – a form of therapeutic massage involving a rhythmic series of finger pressures over the entire body.

Testosterone – an androgen hormone produced by the adrenal cortex, the testes (in men) and the ovaries and adrenal glands (in women). Women with low testosterone levels may experience low libido, depression, fatigue and/or cognitive difficulties. Levels are often low during the menopause.

Urinary incontinence – the involuntary release of urine from the bladder.

Yoga – an ancient spiritual practice from India that aims to tone the mind, body and soul through various moving and static poses and exercises, breathing exercises, diet and meditation.

USEFUL CONTACTS

Liz Earle Wellbeing

Website specialising in accessible and inspiring ways to look good and feel better. Sign up for free regular wellbeing newsletters, including advice on natural remedies and recipes for the menopause.

www.lizearlewellbeing.com

Menopause Doctor

Helpful website run by leading expert and menopause doctor, Dr Louise Newson. With a particular interest in managing the menopause, she feels passionately that women should be offered the correct information about treatment options so they can make informed choices. Dr Newson's private clinic is at the Spire Parkway Hospital, Solihull, Birmingham.

www.menopausedoctor.co.uk

John Studd Women's Health Clinic

Specialist website of Professor John Studd, past chairman of the British Menopause Society and a leading consultant gynaeocologist who runs the private London PMS and Menopause Clinic, as well as the Osteoporosis Screening Centre at 46 Wimpole Street, London W1G 8SD

www.studd.co.uk

Hormone Health

This was founded by Nick Panay and is a private women's health clinic located in London's Harley Street. Hormone Health's team of consultants and associates are specialists in providing women with tailored management of their sexual, reproductive and post-reproductive health.

www.hormonehealth.co.uk

NICE

The National Institute for Health and Care Excellence has a website with a section devoted to the Diagnosis and Management of the Menopause.

www.nice.org.uk

The Daisy Network

Supports those affected by premature menopause. It provides information regarding menopause stages and treatments.

www.daisynetwork.org.uk

British Menopause Society

Provides education, information and guidance to healthcare professionals specialising in all aspects of post-reproductive health.

www.thebms.org.uk

Faculty of Sexual & Reproductive Healthcare of the Royal College of Obstetricians & Gynaecologists

Has useful guidelines regarding contraception in the over-forties.

www.fsrh.org

National Osteoporosis Society
Can help you with the most up-to-date information and advice regarding osteoporosis.

www.nos.org.uk

Bladder Matters
Provides detailed descriptions of pelvic-floor exercises and bladder training.

www.bladdermatters.co.uk

Continence Foundation
A useful source of information regarding current practice and advice on continence.

www.continence-foundation.org.uk

YES
Makes natural personal lubricants, moisturisers and washes for intimate wellbeing.

www.yesyesyes.org

Sylk
Makes natural personal lubricants, moisturisers and washes for intimate wellbeing. Free samples available on request.

www.sylk.co.uk

British Acupuncture Council
The UK's largest professional body for the practice of traditional acupuncture.

www.acupuncture.org.uk

British Wheel of Yoga

Can help you find a yoga teacher in your area from its list. Every person on it has been properly trained (usually 500 teaching hours over three years) and all their courses and those of their accredited groups have to meet stringent quality standards.

www.bwy.org.uk

National Institute of Medical Herbalists

The leading body representing herbal practitioners, can help find a qualified herbalist near you.

www.nimh.org.uk

British Nutrition Foundation

Advice on the right diet to help you during the menopause.

www.nutrition.org.uk

Beat – Beating Eating Disorders

A charity that provides help, support and information for all individuals affected by eating disorders.

www.b-eat.co.uk

Carers UK

Organisation devoted to making life better for people caring for loved ones.

www.carersuk.org

Walking for Health

Provides a countrywide network of groups of people to walk with. It's fantastic if you are single, newly widowed, have a partner who doesn't like walking or if you just don't have a dog!

www.walkingforhealth.org.uk